9-7-2010

# A Statistical Validation of Raindrop Technique®

## David Stewart, PhD

This Research was Supported by
The Center for Aromatherapy Research and Education
who would like to thank Jacquelyn Close, RA
for critically reviewing the manuscript and
contributing several days of voluntary assistance
to help tabulate the data from the forms of this survey.
This report was first published in 2002
under the title of "*The Raindrop Study.*"

Published by
Care Publications
Marble Hill, Missouri
www.carepublications.net

Distributed by
Center for Aromatherapy Research and Education, Inc. (CARE)
RR. 4, Box 646 • Marble Hill, MO 63764
www.RaindropTraining.com
(800) 758-8629
careclasses@raindroptraining.com

ISBN10 0-934426-38-4
ISBN13 978-0-934426-38-1
Library of Congress Control Number
LCCN 2003094676

1st prtg October 2002, 1500 copies
2nd prtg July 2003, 3000 copies
3rd prtg September 2009, 3000 copies

# Table of Contents

Abstract . . . . . . . . . . . . . . . . . . . . . . . . . . . . . . . . . . . . . . . . . . . . 1

**What is Raindrop Technique?** . . . . . . . . . . . . . . . . . . . . . . . . . . . . 3

    Definition of Therapeutic Grade Oil . . . . . . . . . . . . . . . . . . . . . . . 4

    The Need for Research . . . . . . . . . . . . . . . . . . . . . . . . . . . . . . . . . 4

    The Essential Oils Used in Raindrop . . . . . . . . . . . . . . . . . . . . . . 6

    Where Raindrop Gets its Name . . . . . . . . . . . . . . . . . . . . . . . . . . 7

**Research Methodology** . . . . . . . . . . . . . . . . . . . . . . . . . . . . . . . . 9

**Demographics and Research Results** . . . . . . . . . . . . . . . . . . . . . . 11

**Tabulation of Respondent Comments** . . . . . . . . . . . . . . . . . . . . . 21

**Discussion & Conclusion** . . . . . . . . . . . . . . . . . . . . . . . . . . . . . . 51

**Bibliography** . . . . . . . . . . . . . . . . . . . . . . . . . . . . . . . . . . . . . . . 53

**Appendix: Raindrop Survey Questionnaire** . . . . . . . . . . . . . . . . 54

**Index of Conditions Reported by Respondents** . . . . . . . . . . . . . 60

# Abstract

During the past fifteen years, Raindrop Technique has become a widely used therapeutic protocol throughout the United States. Numerous anecdotal accounts relate the significant and substantive benefits generated by this procedure. Raindrop Technique has been use to ameloriate cases of viral infection, kyphosis, scoliosis, chronic fatigue syndrome, and many other conditions.

As its popularity and usage have increased, a small group of aromatherapists has questioned the use of the procedure and its reliance on undiluted therapeutic-grade essential oils. So, in an effort to statistically validate the benefit (or lack thereof) of the Raindrop Technique, I circulated a questionnaire in late 2001 among several thousand aromatherapists, health practitioners, and users of essential oils to poll those who receive Raindrop and those who perform it. This study summarizes the experiences of more than 14,000 sessions of Raindrop.

Of the 422 adults who responded to the survey, 370 were female and 52 were male. They represented 39 states of the United States, 5 provinces of Canada, and 5 other countries. 265 were facilitators, 259 were both facilitators and receivers, 157 were receivers only. Among the 416 receivers, a total of 3,584 Raindrop procedures were experienced (mean value = 8.6 treatments each). Among the 265 facilitators, a total of 11,256 procedures were reported (mean value = 42.5 each). Receivers reported their Raindrop experiences to be Positive (97%), Pleasant (98%), Resulted in healing (16%), Felt better afterwards (98%), Improved health (89%), and Improved emotional state (86%). 99.9% of receivers said they would receive Raindrop again.

The differences in the response rates among those who reported improved health vs. actual healing can be due to the subjects' likely interpretation of the question. "Healing" implies a total resolution of a preexisting disease or health condition, whereas "improved health" merely indicates an improvement (whether slight or great) in health or preexisting condition.

46.2% identified themselves as licensed professionals. 27% were massage therapists (LMT, CMT, RMT). 11% were registered nurses while 1.5% were chiropractors. There was one M.D. and one D.O. who responded.

As for negative responses: 1 in 168 (67 incidences out 11,256 reported Raindrops) considered Raindrop to be unpleasant. 1 in 489 considered it a negative experience. Only 1 in 1,023 said they would not receive Raindrop again. Unpleasant experiences reported (in order of frequency) were: Burning sensation on skin, Skin rashes, Nausea, Headaches, Tiredness. Most identified these as symptoms of a detoxification process. All of these were reported as temporary, often followed by positive results including relief of various symptoms.

Perceived benefits reported (in order of frequency) were: Removed back pain, Stopped cold or flu, Euphoria, Felt energized, Relieved stress or anxiety, General reduction of pain.

The study includes 74 brief commentaries by Raindrop facilitators and receivers that provide insights into the technique, its practice and outcomes, that cannot be discerned from numerical data alone.

# What is Raindrop Technique®?

Raindrop Technique is a procedure for applying essential oils to the feet, back, and spine. It is a form of aromatherapy. It was developed during the 1980s by a naturopathic physician, D. Gary Young. In developing the methodology, Young worked with a Lakota elder. Raindrop incorporates certain Native American concepts, including a special form of massage called "feather stroking" which is similar to a massage technique called "effleurage."[1,2]

Another aspect of Raindrop is "Vita Flex," a therapeutic maneuver adapted from Oriental acupuncture, acupressure, and reflexology. The term, "Vita Flex," meaning "vitality through the reflexes," was coined by Stanley Burroughs, who studied Oriental medicine and brought the technique to the West.[3] Vita Flex involves the gentle pressing and rolling of the Raindrop facilitator's fingertips upon the Raindrop receiver's body surface at specific meridians, or reflex points. The theory of Vita Flex utilizes the fact that the human skin is piezoelectric.[4] That is, when even a slight pressure is applied to the body surface, a voltage is generated, and electric charges move accordingly. The currents so generated are thought to be of therapeutic value.[1,2,3]

Throughout this report, the person performing Raindrop is referred to as the "facilitator" while the one receiving the Raindrop is referred to as the "client" or the "receiver."

In summary, Raindrop Technique is a combination of various aspects of conventional massage, adaptations of Oriental acupressure and reflexology (Vita Flex), Native American healing techniques, and aromatherapy using therapeutic-grade essential oils (defined on the next page). The techniques of Raindrop performed with non-therapeutic grade oils (food or perfume grades) is not a true representation of the method.

## Definition of Therapeutic Grade Oil

A therapeutic grade essential oil is defined here as one that is specially distilled from plants that are grown wild or cultivated organically. Plants should be from the proper botanical genus, species, and cultivar. No chemical fertilizers are added to the soil, and crop cultivation is free of herbicides and pesticides. Plants should be extracted by steam distillation at minimum temperatures and pressures, as was done in ancient times. No chemical solvents are used in the extraction process. Moreover, distillation, condensation, and separation should be performed in vessels constructed of relatively inert materials, such as food-grade stainless steel or glass.

The essential oil must be distilled using low-pressure, low-temperature steam for the proper length of time to ensure that a complete essential oil is extracted, and that there is no significant loss or exclusion of lighter fractions (ie., monoterpenes) or heavier fractions (ie., diterpenes) from the oil.

Finally, the chemical profile of the principal constituents in the oil must fall within the parameters of certain standards such as AFNOR (*Association Francaise de Normalization*) and/or ISO (International Standards Organization). There are, as yet, no standards for therapeutic-grade essential oils set by any government agency in North America.

Therapeutic-grade essential oil should be bottled as it comes from the still, with none of its natural constituents removed and with nothing added. The container and its lid, or seal, must be non-reactive, air tight, and a shield from light, such as bottles of brown, amber, or blue glass.

It should be noted that the vast majority of essential oils (over 90%) are produced for the flavor and fragrance industries and do not fulfill therapeutic standards.[6,9,10,12] Such oils are not considered suitable for use in Raindrop Technique.

## The Need for Research

Raindrop Technique is a procedure that has been performed by thousands of facilitators on many thousands of people since the 1980s throughout the United States, Canada, and in many other countries. There are numerous training programs on the technique, as well as a number of videos and books that describe it. New publications discussing Raindrop seem to emerge every year. Its popularity appears to be growing.

A recent search of the internet using Google and Yahoo search engines produced a list of over 5000 hits for the phrases "raindrop therapy," "raindrop training," and/or "Raindrop Technique." Evidence for the growing interest in receiving and doing Raindrop is suggested by statistical item 10 on page 13 of this report. Of the 416 respondents receiving Raindrop, only 2.5% received their first one before 1996 and only 10% before 1998 while 90% received their first Raindrop since 1998.

This trend is further corroborated by item 14 on page 14 of this report, which has to do with the numbers of Raindrop facilitators being trained and beginning their practices. Out of 265 facilitators who responded to the survey, only 3.8% were trained and began performing the technique before 1996 and only 11% before 1998, while 89% started since 1998.

It is also interesting to note that of the 265 Raindrop facilitators who responded, 46% have a professional license of some kind. 27% were licensed, registered, or certified massage therapists, 11% registered nurses, and 1.5% chiropractors. There was also one MD, one DO, and 10 NDs who reported themselves as performing Raindrop Technique.

Against the background of an expanding demand and interest in Raindrop, there appears to be few, if any, scientific studies as to its theoretical basis or its outcomes. Numerous compilations of personal testimonies, representing hundreds of cases, are available from many sources. No statistical studies appear to have been published to date. This study is the first attempt to supply statistical information on Raindrop outcomes that goes beyond the many collections of anecdotes that currently circulate among those who use essential oils.

It is hoped that the findings of this survey will offer the beginning of a statistical basis for health care professionals, health insurance carriers, massage therapists, aromatherapists, and others to consider the pros and cons of Raindrop. It is also hoped that this study will be a catalyst for many Raindrop studies yet to come.

In addition, it is the intent of this publication to provide a partial basis for informed consent for individuals who wish to consider Raindrop Technique for their own purposes. Additional information for a more fully informed consent is normally provided to the client by the facilitator

## The Essential Oils Used in Raindrop Technique

A typical Raindrop procedure takes about one hour to perform during which seven single essential oils and three blends of essential oils are applied neat to the skin (without dilution). Following the application of the oils, a warm damp towel (layered between two dry towels) is placed on the receiver's back for 5–10 minutes as they rest. Raindrop is usually done on a massage table, although it can be performed in a bed, on a couch, or in a seated position on a chair.

Essential oils are the lipid-soluble portion of the oleo-gum-resins that circulate in plants. They can be extracted in various ways. Those used in Raindrop Technique are extracted by steam distillation.[1,2] The molecules of essential oils are all very small (less than 500 amu) and are, thus, volatile, aromatic, and capable of transdermal absorption by the human body.[5-12]

The single pure essential oils used in Raindrop Technique are as follows:
Basil (*Ocimum basilicum*)
Birch (*Betula alleghaniensis)* *
Cypress (*Cupressus sempervirens*)
Marjoram (*Origanum majorana*)
Oregano (*Origanum vulgare*)
Peppermint (*Mentha piperita*)
Thyme (*Thymus vulgaris*)

* Wintergreen (*Galtheria procumbens*) is often used in place of Birch, the two oils being interchangeable in performing Raindrop Technique.[1,2]

In addition to the above singles, the following blends of oils are also routinely applied in Raindrop Technique:

Blend #1. (Trade name, Valor™)  Blue Tansy (*Tanacetum annuum*), Frankincense (*Boswellia carteri*), Rosewood (*Aniba rosaeodora*), and Spruce (*Picea mariana*) blended with the fatty oil of Almond.[1,2]

Blend #2. (Trade name, Aroma Seiz™)  Basil (*Ocimum basilicum*), Cypress (*Cupressus sempervirens*), Lavender (*Lavandula angustifolia*), Marjoram (*Origanum marjorana*), and Peppermint (*Mentha piperita*).[1,2]

Blend #3. (Trade name, Ortho Ease™) Wintergreen (*Galtheria procumbens*) or Birch (*Betula alleghaniensis*), Eucalyptus (*Eucalyptus ericifolia*), Juniper (*Juniperus osteosperma/scopulorum*), Lemongrass (*Cymbopogon flexuosus*), Marjoram (*Origanum majorana*), Peppermint (*Mentha piperita*), Red Thyme (*Thymus serpyllum*), and Vetiver (*Vetiveria zizanioides*) blended with these fatty oils: Wheatgerm, Grapeseed, Sweet Almond, Olive, and Vitamin E.[1,2]

## Where Raindrop Gets its Name

During portions of the Raindrop procedure, essential oils are dropped neat (undiluted) on the back along the spine from a height of about six inches. This is where the technique gets its name.

The theory of dropping the oils in this manner is that the oils, which are said to possess electromagnetic properties, are allowed to fall through the electromagnetic field of the receiver before touching the skin.[1,2,4] Thus, the oils are thought to interact with the receiver's electric fields in a possibly beneficial way before being absorbed by the body through the skin.

The electrical nature of the Vita Flex maneuver is also thought to assist in the body's absorption and utilization of essential oils.[1,2]

# Research Methodology

As mentioned in the introduction, Raindrop is a technique conceived and developed by D. Gary Young since the 1980s. Young is the founder and owner of a network marketing company known as Young Living Essential Oils, Inc. (YLEO), headquartered in Lehi, Utah. Young has been the principal teacher and disseminator of the Raindrop protocol for many years. Since 1995 he has developed a group of trained instructors that also teach the technique. These YLEO instructors teach what are known as YLEO Level I classes throughout the United States and Canada. These classes have trained thousands who are, almost exclusively, YLEO distributors.

The technique mandates the use of only pure, unadulterated, therapeutic grade essential oils. Since there are few brands of oils in North America that meet these standards in a way that is easily verified, Raindrop Technique is principally a methodology practiced by YLEO distributors or by people who use YLEO oils exclusively to be assured of their quality. Therefore, by necessity, at this time a study of Raindrop Technique means that almost all of the participants will be associated with YLEO in some way.

In fact, out of 256 facilitators who responded to the survey, only eight (3.1%) said they used oils other than those of YLEO to perform Raindrop. (See statistical item 16 on p. 18.) Two respondents (other than the eight) said they had tried other brands of oils for Raindrop, but for various reasons had ceased doing so and now used only YLEO oils. Five of the eight (62.5%) said they used mostly YLEO oils, but occasionally used other brands as well. Two said they used only YLEO oils except for birch, which they got from another supplier when YLEO discontinued carrying this oil. Only one of the eight said they used mostly other brands of oils, but even this individual also used the YLEO brand as well. Hence, every facilitator responding to this survey used YLEO oils to one degree or another in doing Raindrop, 96.9% of them exclusively.

The results of the eight questionnaires including oils other than the YLEO brand were all strongly on the positive side and statistically the same as the overall results of the survey. That is, their inclusion or exclusion did not significantly alter any of the final figures. Hence, all eight are included in the tabulations that follow.

During October, November, and December, 2001, a Raindrop survey questionnaire was distributed to several email chat lines. (See Appendix A for the complete content of the questionnaire.) During the span of time the questionnaire was being circulated, it was posted several times to each chat line. In consideration of the foregoing facts, all but one of these chat lines were mainly composed of YLEO distributors. The eight chatlines to which the survey was posted are as follows:

Aromatherapy@idma.com
AromatherapyOils@yahoogroups.com
EssentialOilers@yahoogroups.com
EssOils@yahoogroups.com
HealthLineOnLine@yahoogroups.com
JOYgroup@yahoogroups.com
OilFountain@yahoogroups.com
PineHillGroup@yahoogroups.com

In addition, a number of YLEO leaders with extensive email lists of their own publicized the questionnaire among their YLEO Affiliates while other leaders made hard copies that were handed or mailed out. The actual number of people who received the questionnaire is unknown and undeterminable, but may well be in excess of 2,000–3,000. The number completing and returning the survey is 422. Even if the survey reached 4,000 people, 422 is better than a 10% return.

Aromatherapy@idma.com was composed almost entirely of non-YLEO distributors. Although there were negative comments on Raindrop Technique among the members of this chat line that continued throughout the last quarter of 2001, only one questionnaire could be identified as having originated from that source. The scant response from this chatline was due to the fact that there was a refusal to cooperate in any way with this study, which seemd odd given that this study would have been an ideal forum to expose any hazards or limitations of Raindrop. In actual fact, their lack of any first-hand experience with Raindrop Technique would have disqualified them as candidates for this survey regardless of their boycott, especially since opinions and conjecture are not sufficient to generate reliable data for a study of this nature.

# Demographics and Research Results

The Questionnaire from which the following statistics were obtained is given in Appendix A. The results are organized and numbered in twenty-one parts.

1. **Total Respondents:** ................................ 422

2. **Gender of Respondents:**
   Female ................................... 370  (87.6%)
   Male ..................................... 52  (12.4%)

3. **General Geographic Distribution:**
   U.S.A. ...................................391  (92.7%)
   (from 39 states, Puerto Rico, and D.C.)
   Canada .....................................25  (5.9%)
   (from five provinces)
   Other Countries ............................ 6  (1.4%)
   (from five different nations)

4. **U.S. Distribution by State (391 total):**

   | | | | |
   |---|---|---|---|
   | Alabama | 2 | Nebraska | 2 |
   | Arizona | 9 | New Jersey | 20 |
   | Arkansas | 1 | New York | 40 |
   | California | 89 | New Mexico | 4 |
   | Colorado | 24 | North Carolina | 4 |
   | Connecticut | 1 | North Dakota | 1 |
   | Delaware | 1 | Ohio | 11 |
   | Dist. of Columbia | 1 | Oklahoma | 12 |
   | Florida | 9 | Oregon | 16 |
   | Georgia | 1 | Pennsylvania | 7 |
   | Hawaii | 1 | Puerto Rico | 1 |
   | Illinois | 5 | South Carolina | 4 |
   | Indiana | 6 | South Dakota | 4 |
   | Iowa | 10 | Tennessee | 3 |
   | Louisiana | 2 | Texas | 5 |
   | Maryland | 5 | Utah | 3 |
   | Massachusetts | 3 | Vermont | 1 |
   | Michigan | 7 | Virginia | 4 |
   | Minnesota | 8 | Washington | 5 |
   | Missouri | 52 | West Virginia | 2 |
   | Montana | 5 | | |

5. **Canadian Distribution by Province (25 total):**

| | | | |
|---|---|---|---|
| Alberta | 8 | Ontario | 5 |
| British Columbia | 10 | Saskatchewan | 1 |
| Quebec | 1 | | |

6. **Distribution by Other Countries (6 total):**

| | | | |
|---|---|---|---|
| Australia | 2 | Sweden | 1 |
| Japan | 1 | West Indies | 1 |
| Netherlands | 1 | | |

7. **Relationships of Respondents to Raindrop**
   **422 (100%) had either received or performed (facilitated) at least one Raindrop**
   265 (62.6%) were facilitators
       (i.e. they had administered at least one Raindrop)
   6 (1.4%) were facilitators only
       (i.e. they had performed Raindrop but had never received one)
   259 (61.4%) were both receivers and facilitators
       (i.e. They had both performed and received Raindrop)
   157 (37.2%) were clients only
       (i.e. they had received but never facilitated)

8. **Total Raindrops Received:** 3,584
   (received by 416 clients, Mean value = 8.6 Raindrop procedures per respondent receiver)

9. **Number of Times Received by Respondent**

| | Number of Recipients | |
|---|---|---|
| 1 time | 76 | (18.27%) |
| 2-3 times | 108 | (25.96%) |
| 4-5 times | 75 | (18.03%) |
| 6-10 times | 70 | (16.83%) |
| 11-20 times | 46 | (11.06%) |
| 21-30 times | 22 | (5.29%) |
| 31-50 times | 3 | (3.13%) |
| 51-80 times | 5 | (1.20%) |
| more than 80 | 1 | (0.24%) |

(percents based on 416 receivers)

10. **Year When Respondent First Received Raindrop:**

Number of Recipients

Before 1994 ................................. 1   (0.24%)
1994–1995 ................................. 9   (2.16%)
1996–1997 ................................. 32  (7.69%)
1998–1999 ................................. 129 (31.01%)
2000–2001 ................................. 245 (58.89%)

(percents shown based on 416 receivers)

11. **Perceived Results of Raindrop as Expressed by 416 clients receiving 3,584 Raindrops:**

| | | | |
|---|---|---|---|
| a. | Positive<br>97.0% | Neutral<br>2.5% | Negative<br>0.5% |
| b. | Pleasant<br>97.9% | Neutral<br>1.4% | Unpleasant<br>0.4% |
| c. | Resulted in<br>Healing<br>15.9% | No Perceptible<br>Results<br>83.9% | Resulted in<br>Harm or Injury<br>0.2% |
| d. | Felt Better<br>Afterwards<br>97.7% | No Change<br>in Feeling<br>1.4% | Felt Worse<br>Afterwards<br>0.9% |
| e. | Health<br>Improved<br>89.1% | No Change<br>in Health<br>10.9% | Health got<br>Worse<br>0.0% |
| f. | Emotional State<br>Improved<br>86.2% | No Change<br>in Emotions<br>13.4% | Emotional State<br>Worsened<br>0.4% |
| g. | Would Receive<br>It Again<br>99.9% | Maybe So<br>Maybe Not<br>0.1% | Would Never<br>Receive it Again<br>0.0% |

12. **Total Raindrops Administered:** 11,256
(performed by 265 facilitators, Mean value = 42.5 Raindrop
procedures per respondent facilitator)

13. **Number of Times Performed by Facilitator**

| | Number of Facilitators | |
|---|---|---|
| 1 time | 14 | (5.30%) |
| 2-3 times | 25 | (9.47%) |
| 4-5 times | 26 | (9.85%) |
| 6-10 times | 44 | (16.7%) |
| 11-20 times | 41 | (15.5%) |
| 21-30 times | 31 | (11.7%) |
| 31-50 times | 33 | (12.5%) |
| 51-100 times | 23 | (8.71%) |
| 101-200 times | 24 | (9.10%) |
| 102-400 times | 2 | (0.76%) |
| more than 400 | 1 | (0.38%) |

(percents based on 265 facilitators)

14. **Year When Facilitator First Performed Raindrop:**

| | Number of Facilitators | |
|---|---|---|
| Before 1994 | 2 | (0.76%) |
| 1994–1995 | 8 | (3.03%) |
| 1996–1997 | 20 | (7.58%) |
| 1998-1999 | 82 | (31.1%) |
| 2000-2001 | 152 | (57.6%) |

(percents based on 265 facilitators)

15. How Facilitators Received Their Training
(Note: Most were trained from more than one source)

   A. Where Hands-On Training Was Received:
   Attended Young Living Essential Oils Level I . . . . . . .149  (56.4%)
   Taught by Someone Who Took YLEO Level I . . . . .114  (43.2%)
   Received Training from Mindful Healing Center . . .118  (44.7%)
   One-on-one or small group with D. Gary Young, ND . . 33  (12.5%)
   CARE Classes . . . . . . . . . . . . . . . . . . . . . . . . . . . . . 31  (11.7%)

   Young Living Essential Oils
     3125 W. Executive Parkway, Lehi, UT 84043
   Mindful Healing Center, 6005 W. Miller Rd., Ste. #6
     Schwartz Creek, MI 48507
   CARE = Center for Aromatherapy Research & Education
     Rt. 4, Box 646, Marble Hill, MO 63764

   B. Raindrop Training Books That Were Used:
   (See Bibliography for more complete information)
   *Essential Oils Desk Reference*, Brian Manwaring, Editor
   Essential Science Publishing, Orem, UT. 461 pp.
   • Used by 153 facilitators surveyed (58.0%)
   *Aromatherapy: The Essential Beginning*, by Gary Young,
   Essential Press Publishing, Salt Lake City, UT 174 pp.
   • Used by 2 facilitators surveyed (0.76%)
   *Reference Guide for Essential Oils*, by Connie and Alan
   Higley, Abundant Health, Olathe, KS. 497 pp.
   • Used by 4 facilitators surveyed (1.52%)

   C. Raindrop Training Videos That Were Used:
   Videos with Raindrop Demonstrated by Gary Young (4 such videos)
   • Used by 100 facilitators surveyed (37.9%)
   Video with Raindrop Demonstrated by David Stewart
   • Used by 49 facilitators surveyed (18.6%)
   Video with Raindrop Demonstrated by Cathy Eaton
   • Used by 23 facilitators surveyed (8.71%
   Video with Raindrop Demonstrated by Jeri Bocci
   * Used by 10 facilitators surveyed (3.79%)
   (percents above based on 265 facilitators)

## 16. Oil Brands for Doing Raindrop Technique Used by Facilitators Responding to this Survey.

Facilitators Using YLEO Oils Exclusively ........ 256 (96.97%)

Facilitators Using YLEO Oils Exclusively
(Except for Birch Oil) ....................... 2 (0.76%)

Facilitators Using YLEO Oils Mostly,
Who Occasionally Use Other Brands ........... 5 (1.89%)

Facilitators Using Other Brands Mostly,
Who Occasionally Use YLEO Oils ............. 1 (0.38%)

(Percents based on 265 facilitators)

NOTE: In addition to the non-YLEO oils used by the eight facilitators tabulated above, two facilitators responding to the survey said they had formerly used other brands but now use only YLEO oils. One of these (a Licensed Massage Therapist from South Carolina) said: "Other brands I have tried in the past burn the skin and dry it." The other (a Registered Nurse from Oregon) said: "I have used other oils, but will no longer do that because the purity/integrity of many are in question for me. I base this on experiences I've had with some lavenders probably with high camphor levels that should not have been in the oil as it was advertised. Due to these experiences I will not use any oils other than YLEO. For me the integrity of the system prior to the production of an oil is important. I know if I use a Young Living oils I don't need to wonder what I have in my hands. I know I have a therapeutic-grade oil, not an oil that says that it is and has dangerous solvents, etc., in the same bottle. The purity/integrity of the oil used in Raindrop is critical and more important than the technique."

## 17. Professional Credentials of Facilitators, as Reported on the Questionnaire

### A. Professional vs. Nonprofessional Status

Licensed Professional (i.e. recognized in
some capacity by a government licensing agency) ...122   (46.2%)
Not a Licensed Professional ...................142   (53.4%)

### B. Facilitator Specialties Identified:

Of the 142 without a license, about half of these reported holding
certifications or degrees related to the healing arts.

Massage Therapist (LMT, CMT, RMT) .......... 72   (27.3%)
Registered Nurse (RN) ....................... 29   (11.0%)
Reiki Master/Instructor ...................... 15   (5.68%)
Beautician, Cosmetologist, Esthetician .......... 11   (4.17%)
Doctor of Naturopathy (ND) ................. 10   (3.79%)
Certified CARE Instructor (CCI) .............. 10   (3.79%)
Licensed Practical Nurse (LPN) .................6   (2.27%)
Natural/Holistic Health Practitioner ............ 6   (2.27%)
Licensed Counselor/Psychotherapist ............ 5   (1.89%)
Registered Aromatherapist (RA) ............... 5   (1.89%)
Healing Touch, Touch for Health, etc.  ......... 5   (1.89%)
Doctor of Chiropractic (DC) .................. 4   (1.52%)
Ordained or Licensed Minister/Priest ............ 4   (1.52%)
Various Doctors of Philosophy (PhD) ............ 3   (1.14%)
Physical Therapist (LPT, RPT) ..................2   (0.76%)
Licensed Social Worker ...................... 2   (0.76%)
Cert. Natural Health Pract'ner (CNHP) .......... 2   (0.76%)
Certified Reflexologist (CR) .................. 2   (0.76%)
Certified Acupuncturist ...................... 2   (0.76%)
Registered Engineer (RE, PE) ................. 2   (0.76%)
Doctor of Medicine (MD) .................... 1   (0.38%)
Doctor of Osteopathy (DO) .................... 1   (0.38%)
Doctor of Healing Arts ...................... 1   (0.38%)
Asian Body Therapist ....................... 1   (0.38%)
Licensed Audiologist ......................... 1   (0.38%)
Plus one each of several unknown acronyms such as
DPM, LSCC, RDH, RNP, RHY, RPP, TFA

18. Perceived Results of Raindrop as Expressed by Clients to the 265 Facilitators Responding to this Survey for 11,256 Raindrop Procedures Administered:

| | | | |
|---|---|---|---|
| a, | Positive<br>96.3% | Neutral<br>3.5% | Negative<br>0.2% |
| b. | Pleasant<br>96.4% | Neutral<br>3.0% | Unpleasant<br>0.6% |
| c. | Resulted in<br>Healing<br>87.7% | No Perceptible<br>Results<br>12.0% | Resulted in<br>Harm or Injury<br>0.3% |
| d. | Felt Better<br>Afterwards<br>96.0% | No Change<br>in Feeling<br>3.4% | Felt Worse<br>Afterwards<br>0.6% |
| e. | Health<br>Improved<br>90.8% | No Change<br>in Health<br>9.2% | Health got<br>Worse<br>0.03% |
| f. | Emotional State<br>Improved<br>91.0% | No Change<br>in Emotions<br>8.5% | Emotional State<br>Worsened<br>0.5% |
| g. | Would Receive<br>It Again<br>96.7% | Maybe So<br>Maybe Not<br>3.2% | Would Never<br>Receive it Again<br>0.1% |

19. Summary of Negative Responses Given Above:

Considered Raindrop a Negative Experience  . . . . . . . . 1 in 489
    23 incidences
Considered Raindrop to be Unpleasant . . . . . . . . . . . . 1 in 168
    67 incidences
Felt Raindrop Caused Harm or Injury  . . . . . . . . . . . . 1 in 331
    34 incidences
Felt Worse after Raindrop  . . . . . . . . . . . . . . . . . . . . . . 1 in 165
    68 incidences
Felt State of Health got Worse  . . . . . . . . . . . . . . . . . . 1 in 3,752
    3 incidences

Felt Emotional State was Worse . . . . . . . . . . . . . . . . . . 1 in 201
    56 incidences
Would Never Receive a Raindrop Again . . . . . . . . . . 1 in 1,023
    11 incidences

20. **Unpleasant Experiences Reported:**
(Listed in order of frequency, the first being the most
frequently mentioned)
  1. Burning sensation on the skin
  2. Skin Rashes
  3. Nausea
  4. Headaches
  5. Tiredness afterwards

21. **Perceived Benefits Reported:**
(Listed in order of frequency, the first being the most
frequently mentioned)
  1. Removed back pain
  2. Stopped cold or flu
  3. Euphoria
  4. Felt energized
  5. Relieved stress or anxiety
  6. General reduction of pain

A sample of other perceived benefits reported (not in any particular order):
  Experienced detoxification
  Correction of scoliosis
  Relief of sciatica
  Lower blood pressure
  Relief from arthritis
  Helped alleviate migraines or recurring headaches
  Lowered cholesterol
  Helped insomnia
  Relief of allergies
  Relief of asthma and respiratory congestion
  Relief from depression
  Increased bodily movement
  Mitigated side effects of chemotherapy
  (See pp. 21-49 for more details)

# Tabulation of Respondent Comments

Among the 422 questionnaires returned, there are hundreds of comments and testimonials. To reprint all of them would require a large book. Those selected here are representative of what was received. The comments include not only testimonials of benefits from Raindrop, but problems, untoward effects, and suggestions for their solutions as provided by the responders to this survey. They do not necessarily represent the opinions or policies of the Center for Aromatherapy Research and Education, nor those of the author. They are not to be construed as making any claims for the results of Raindrop Technique nor for any particular brand of essential oil but are only presented as data obtained by this survey. None of these statements have been independently confirmed by a qualified, independent researcher. They are reproduced here for educational and research purposes only to provide insights that cannot be communicated by mere statistics. These comments should be interpreted within the limitations of their origin. They are not intended for purposes of diagnosing, prescribing, or treating any disease, illness, or injured condition of the body. The author, publisher, and printer accept no responsibility for such use. Anyone suffering from any disease, illness, or injury should consult with a physician or other appropriate licensed health care professional.

The sources of the foregoing comments are all confidential, identified only by a state, province, country and/or profession. All of these records are on permanent file at the Center for Aromatherapy Research and Education (CARE). With few exceptions, all 422 respondents could be identified from the forms they submitted and could be contacted if such a need was deemed necessary. The confidentiality of the responders was guaranteed when the survey was made—a promise that will be respected and preserved.

## Quadriplegic Raises Arms; Night Sweats Stop

My first experience with Raindrop was convincing. My son, who is a quadriplegic, had frozen shoulders and was unable to raise his arms more than a few inches in spite of daily exercising. During Raindrop, his back noticeably heated and I applied carrier oil. About 15 minutes later, he was able to raise his arms nearly to shoulder height!

The other most memorable experience was a client with a brain tumor which caused the left side of his face to be nearly paralyzed. During Raindrop his neck and shoulders heated. The following week he came to see me and was very excited. For four years since the operation, he had terrible night sweats that left the bed linens stained and had a rank odor. After the Raindrop, his sweats had ceased. His wife confirmed. Now, after three years, he still has none of these sweats.

— *Licensed Acupressure Massage Therapist, South Carolina*

## Out of Pain and Two Inches Taller

I have had scoliosis since I was eleven years old, when I grew five inches in three months. It really did not start creating any problems until it reached a 55° curve at about 42 years of age. I was in constant pain in my back and it was pulling my right knee inward causing it a great deal of pain. It also took the natural curve out of my neck. This all started in my mid-thirties. I am now 47.

A year-and-a-half ago a naturopathic doctor friend of mine introduced me to the Raindrop Technique. After four treatments done within one month I was out of pain and two inches taller. My curve is now backed down to 42°. The oils have become a way of life for my family and me. I will continue the Raindrops for myself and my family because it works.

— *Scoliosis Success in Indiana*

## Standing Monthly Appointment

I have a standing monthly appointment for Raindrop and have received the technique 20 times. I felt like I was doing something very good for my body. I was considering every two weeks instead of once a month. My circulation has improved dramatically, and my feet are no longer cold all the time. If this wonderful technique was ever stopped, I would still find a way to do Raindrop even if it was in my own home.

— *Regular Receiver in Michigan*

## Benefits to a Healthy Person

I am someone in general good health, so I never had specific complaints about chronic stuff. Whenever I have received Raindrop (which is about 15 times now), it was always profoundly relaxing and felt supportive in an overall way. My muscles seemed to relax and I would also experience a general sense of well-being.

— *Certified Massage Therapist in California*

## Blissfully Detoxed

I am a bodyworker and intend to administer Raindrop as soon as I receive the training. I received Raindrop for the first time just last week. I found the experience to be extremely relaxing and emotionally uplifting. I even felt blissful immediately following the treatment.

The Raindrop complimented other treatments I have been having lately for muscle fatigue and spinal maladjustment in my C-spine and T-spine. It's hard to say which therapy has benefited me the most. They are all working together. I would definitely have Raindrop again and will be recommending it to my clients.

There were two negative aspects. (They didn't really bother me, but might someone else.) First, the oils did burn a little bit around C7, T1 . . . upper shoulder area. The therapist and I discussed this. It could be because this is an area where I have been experiencing difficulty lately and I also have a small cyst at C7, T1. She added some vegetable oil to cool it down a bit.

Secondly, I did have some breaking out (irritation rash) along the spine in certain areas the day of and the next day after the treatment. I attributed this to toxins being released. I had my husband apply some evening primrose lotion (Aubrey Organics) and this calmed it down rather quickly.

— *Bodyworker in California*

## Temporary Relief of Foot Pain

After Raindrop my chronic plantar fascitis (pain in the foot) was totally gone for three or four days. I had it for two years with periodic slight improvement. I also felt a healing in general that I can not explain. Slept wonderful for the next couple of nights and that is not my history to sleep well.

— *Slept Wonderful in Colorado*

## No Health Problems, No Dramatic Changes

I have received six Raindrop sessions and am a very healthy person. I didn't come into my RDT sessions with any particular need for healing and so didn't notice any particular change. It was always pleasant.
— *Always Pleasant in Michigan*

## Over-The-Counter Pain Relievers More Dangerous

In 25 years as a health professional I can certainly testify to some dangerous things I've witnessed. I do not count the Raindrop Technique as one of them. Education is definitely important. I was not foolish enough to do Raindrop without training. I do not consider my two extensive days of training my only training, but the many hours of study and my own personal oil use and that of my family's as important ground work as well. I have looked for many years to find something that is complimentary to my beliefs. I do not pretend to be an aromatherapist, just as I did not pretend to be a pharmacist when I used to take an Advil® or a cold preparation. I would never be questioned if I used or gave friends or family an Advil. So why would helping those I care about using Raindrop or oils be a threat to anyone? The reality is that Advil has been more harmful than any oil I have used.
— *Registered Nurse, Oregon*

## Not Unlike Reiki

I received Raindrop Technique twice and both times found it to be extremely pleasant and soothing and to have lasting positive effects of my general health (including specific back pain) and emotional well-being (on one of the occasions I was dealing with the recent death of my father). I think the technique is a very good one. It seemed to me to add to the beneficial properties of the oils a cumulative energetic cleansing/aligning not unlike Reiki.
— *New South Wales, Australia*

## Results Not Dramatic When You're Healthy

Raindrop Technique was relaxing and enjoyable as a massage, yet I didn't perceive any dramatic health or emotional benefits. However, I am not experiencing any intense physical or emotional pain so it is not so easy to observe a difference.
— *No Pain in California*

## From Hopelessness to a New Life

Six months ago I was ready to throw in the towel. I could not walk or sit up without severe, crippling pain. I couldn't sleep, sit at my computer, drive a car, go to the movies, and could not lift anything heavier than my full coffee cup. Of course I couldn't work, so my income, along with my zest for living, had plummeted to zero. Within one day my whole life had changed when the x-ray and MRI diagnosis found that, because of my extreme congenital scoliosis, I had finally worn away the end of a vertebra, and the nerves were exposed. My body had also formed synovial cysts which, according to everything I had read, "these cysts do not resolve by themselves. They tend to get bigger and the only remedy is surgery." My doctor also stated: "These cysts are serious pain generators." Well, I'd second that!

So there I was, flat on my back, eating narcotics, anti-inflammatories, and muscle relaxants, and washing them down with way too much wine. Friends were making arrangements for me to move in with them so they could take care of me. All in all I was a mess, and life was looking pretty grim.

"Well, why not try surgery?" Surgery for the reduction of synovial cysts comes with huge risk factors (total paralysis) so I didn't see that as an option. The other part of the picture is that I do not have health insurance and could not even consider losing all that I have worked so hard for on a surgery that would be questionable at best. I might have ended up in worse condition and totally penniless. So what was next?

Since I was not "living," as I define "living," and I saw no obvious hope, I decided to plan my death. The thought of planning my own passing seemed, under the circumstances, very reasonable. That's how bad I was.

When I shared my desperation with a friend who is an LMT she was speechless. She made me promise not to do anything for a while. A few days later she called and said, "I just went to this workshop and learned this Raindrop Technique for scoliosis so I want to do it on you." My response was anything but positive, but I agreed.

That was six months ago. Today, I am, with few restrictions, after many Raindrop treatments and ongoing use of the oils, totally back to a normal, active existence. Yes, I occasionally still have pain, but it is pain I can manage. And my use of narcotics has dropped from daily multiple usage to a rare need. And then it is only because I felt so good I have overdone! I have not had to take any muscle relaxants since that first Raindrop and have gone from a minimum of twelve anti-inflammatories a day to maybe two.

Happily, I can once again hike 8 to 10 miles, canoe, pull weeds in my garden, sit at my computer, pick up my 30 lb. granddaughter, go to the movies, drive all day, and sleep soundly all because of these very pure, very powerful oils.

— *Registered Nurse and RNP from Oregon*

## Raindrop as a Detox for the Facilitator

As a therapist, when I do as many as four (my most ever) RDT sessions in a day I have noticed some major reactions afterwards. The next day I had rashes in lymph areas, headache, diarrhea and general fatigue. I returned to normal in 24 hours or less. Considering that was a quadruple dose of oils, I felt that it was not a surprising result. The exposure for the therapist is a very effective way of stimulating a cleanse.

— *Auricular Detox Specialist, Michigan*

## Five Positive, One Negative

I am a chiropractor and have received three Raindrops and have done three. All six were pleasant and the outcomes positive except my first one when I got very sick. I missed a week of work. I assume it means that I have a high viral load or, perhaps, the person that worked on me used too much oil. Subsequent Raindrops have not had this effect on me nor, in my limited experience, have I seen it in anyone else.

— *Chiropractor in California*

## Resolved Emotions

I have received Raindrop five times and have done it ten. My very first Raindrop I felt much more energized, afterwards. I didn't feel any pain or discomfort during the procedure, and my husband was the one who administered it by following the directions in the *Essential Oils Desk Reference*, second edition. The last Raindrop I received I experienced a release of pent up emotions that have been buried for quite some time. Following the procedure, I felt energized and the emotion I worked through appeared to be resolved (that was two months ago).

— *Certified Massage Therapist from Illinois*

## Whiplash Injuries

I have received great help from Raindrop in relieving neck and arm pain after a fall off a chair. Chiropractic did not give as much benefit. I continue to have some neck problems since I have had several whiplash injuries in my life, but when I receive the Raindrop, I have no pain for several weeks afterwards. I desire to receive more Raindrops to keep me out of pain.

A friend of mine has back pain which improved for weeks after she received a Raindrop. She has told me that "nothing else has gotten rid of her pain so completely." She wants to continue to get them. We trade sessions with each other on a monthly basis now that we are both trained.

— *Raindrop Partners in California*

## Spinal Meningitis, Epstein-Barr, and Scoliosis

The first person I ever did RDT on was a young lady with viral spinal meningitis. She had had a headache for over a week and was in terrible pain, unable to sleep or rest in any way. The doctor had prescribed pain pills. They did nothing for her, even when she doubled up on them. I gave her a RDT from just reading instructions in a book. She went to sleep during the "event" and slept for two hours. She awakened without a headache for the first time since she'd become ill. She continued to use the oils when she got a headache and soon made a full recovery.

The next person was a lady with Epstein-Barr. She had a series of eight Raindrops and liked them so much that she has recently contacted me and wants another series of eight. She says they give her energy for the coming week. She sleeps better and says "my mind is clearer." Her Epstein-Barr is asymptomatic.

The next person was an 84-year-old man with scoliosis. When I first measured him he was 66.5 inches tall. At the end of the first treatment he was one inch taller. He loves the Raindrop Technique and is still getting one a week. He has been getting them for five months now. His height the last time I measured was 69.75 inches and his back is straight. He still has some atrophied muscles, but is doing exercises to loosen and rebuild them. He loves the oils and uses them faithfully every day on his feet, back, and legs.

— *Retired Nurse in Arizona*

## Sciatic Nerve Pain

I have received two Raindrops, and after the first one I felt intoxicated and light headed for about an hour. I have done about 20 Raindrops on others. On one person her sciatic nerve pain disappeared after the treatment.
— *Raindrop Facilitator in Hawaii*

## Bell's Palsy

Our family has had many good experiences with Raindrop Technique. The most notable was when my husband had Bell's palsy. He came home from work looking like he'd had a stroke. His facial muscles on one side of his face were paralyzed. Everything on that side of his face drooped and his speech was impaired so I couldn't understand anything he said. He also couldn't drink without dribbling. Thankfully, it wasn't a stroke, but it turned out to be Bell's palsy. After learning that it can take weeks or months to get the facial muscles back to normal, I said, "No way! We have oils that will do the job in no time." I looked up Bell's palsy in the book, "Embraced by the Essence." It said that it is thought to be a virus that attacks the facial nerves. We used an oil blend called Thieves™ to kill the virus. We also did Raindrop Technique and added nerve-regenerating oils to help the damaged nerves — Frankincense, Peppermint, Geranium, and Vitex. Within days he was completely recovered. There is no evidence that there was ever a problem.
— *A Wife from Ohio*

## Chronic Back Ache from Scoliosis

When receiving Raindrop I felt my spine has never felt more alive, tingling, and energized. I felt clear headed afterwards with no detox symptoms. It was deeply relaxing and muscularly relieving. I have performed the technique 18 times on others. Most felt deeply relaxed and said "more so than with massage." Several felt a huge reduction in muscle tension. One was alleviated of chronic back ache due to scoliosis for more than a week after the RDT. Many felt very clear headed and extremely energized the next day. Most of them requested to do it again. Only two or three felt worse right afterwards with headache or nausea, but this lasted less than a 24-hour period in all cases.
— *Licensed Massage Therapist in Oregon*

## Scoliosis Corrected

I am not a health care professional, but I have performed Raindrop Technique on others about 21 times and have received the procedure about 20 times myself for scoliosis. The top curve went from 22° to 0° and the bottom curve has gone from 36° to 18°.

— *Raindrop Practitioner, Missouri*

## Pneumonia from Flu Vaccine

Two years ago I received a flu shot where I work as a registered nurse and developed the flu which turned into pneumonia. Over the next several months, after taking antibiotics and doing everything I could to try and get better, I was still tired and run down. At this time I was attending massage therapy classes and I met a friend there who gave me a Raindrop massage. Within two days I could see a difference in my stamina, breathing and energy level. Within a week I felt like a different person.

Throughout the next two years when I would start to come down with a cold, malaise, or when I over-extended myself at work, school or home, I would get a Raindrop. My friend showed me how to do the technique, and in turn, I have helped my sister and friends.

Having the Raindrop helped my body to get back to a homeostasis state naturally, faster, and healthier without having to pay a lot of money to go to the doctor, buy expensive medicines (which have side effects that make me feel worse), and I was able to return to work and school sooner than I had ever done before I discovered Raindrop.

— *Registered Nurse from Tennessee*

## Alleviating Muscle and Nerve Pain

I am a certified aromatherapist and have administered approximately 40 RDTs. Each and every client has stated Raindrop to be effective at alleviating muscle and nerve pain. Not one client has found this to be otherwise. Many have come back wanting to purchase the oils because Raindrop was so effective at ridding cold symptoms, back pain, and, in one case, severe sciatica. There has been no burning or reddening of tissue when the oils were applied neat, and then diluted a minute or two afterwards.

— *Certified Aromatherapist, Alberta, Canada*

## Herniated Disk

My personal experiences with being a receiver of Raindrop Technique have been nothing but wonderful! In February of this year I was suffering with constant low back pain due to what my doctor diagnosed as a herniated disk. I attended a workshop on Raindrop Technique. My husband volunteered to be the receiver as a demonstration of the proper technique. He, too, had had low back pain and some curvature in his upper spine. When she had finished, his spine was markedly straighter, and he felt great relief in his lower back. He said it not only physically helped him, he also had greater mental clarity that lasted for a period of 2–3 weeks.

We purchased a set of Raindrop oils that day and have shared it with many of our friends and relatives since. I have performed the technique about 25 times on twelve different individuals. I am very happy to say that all of them have had very positive results with the Raindrop. No one has ever experienced any negative side effects, rashes, allergic reactions, or the like. The oils, which I apply neat, have never caused any harm to anyone that I have used them on or to whom I personally know who use them. Some have had the most powerful healing happen to them, not only physically, but mentally and spiritually. And I have witnessed that.

And, as for my herniated, disk . . . doesn't bother me a bit any more!
— *Raindrop Facilitator in Ohio*

## Clients in World Trade Center on 9/11/01

I am a licensed massage therapist, and Raindrop is my first choice when a new client comes to me with "everything" wrong. It settles mental and physical stuff to a level that the massage will be more beneficial. Also, some people still come for their massage even if they are sick, like with a cold. I usually will do a Raindrop on them before the massage to help the healing start, as well as clearing the sinuses. Since a lot of my clients were in the World Trade Center on 9/11, they had lots of physical and mental issues when they showed up at my office. I used the Raindrop Technique prior to their massages to induce relaxation and get them to start releasing all that was stored in their muscle tissues. Raindrop just feels fantastic and helps you relax.
— *Licensed Massage Therapist from New Jersey*

## Sinus Infection

Two years ago I had a serious sinus infection which did not respond to antibiotic treatment. What the antibiotics did do was to upset the balance of my flora and cause a yeast infection. My physician (a general practitioner) suggested an option—Raindrop Technique. I was terrified at the idea, knowing my drug (pharmaceutical) sensitivities, but I agreed to do it. Within five minutes of the application of oregano and thyme, my body released so much garbage that I blew my nose for a full five minutes. I wondered where it all came from! Yes, my back was hot and red, but dilution came easily with a mixing oil. My personal feeling is that this reaction was not allergic at all, but the rapid response of my cells being oxygenated and releasing toxins. This was not a burn from fire, but rather heat from energy. Following the session, the activity of the oils continued noticeably for a week, changing lots of body processes—all for the better. I never took my second round of antibiotics, nor have I had any since. I have since received about a dozen RDTs myself and have done five or six on family members with 100% positive results.

— *Grateful for Raindrop in Arkansas*

## Dowager's Hump Almost Disappears

I have received Raindrop ten times and have performed more than fifty. The most dramatic results were when I gave a treatment to a woman with a large dowager's hump. She stood at least two inches taller, and the hump disappeared by 90%. You could hardly see it. She reported to me that her shoulder pain and low back pain was gone and stayed away for three weeks. She enjoys Raindrop Technique very much.

— *Enjoys Raindrop in Puerto Rico*

## Emotional Release Following Raindrop

I personally really enjoyed the Raindrop experience. At first I didn't really notice a big effect like I had heard others talk about. I did notice a decrease in the amount of discomfort I was feeling in my wrists. In fact it was almost gone and about two hours after the experience I became VERY emotional and empathetic. I thought it was REALLY weird. I do not know if Raindrop had anything to do with it or if it had to do with the fact that a few days later I found out that I was pregnant.

— *Unexpectectantly Pregnant in Oregon*

## Releasing Viruses, Emotions, and Toxins

I have no professional health care or massage license, but have been doing Raindrops since 1998 when I was trained in the technique. I have performed the technique 60–70 times. I have seen tremendous physical and emotional changes in people from Raindrop: (1) Many who are prone to colds and bronchitis seemed to present more resistence to infection; those already infected seemed to have faster recovery. (2) Many have released emotions such as grief, fear patterns, etc. (3) Raindrop is a cleansing process for many people for liver, pancreas issues. (4) Many have eliminated back, hip, and neck pain. (5) Almost all people are more relaxed. The only negative I have seen is slight nausea if someone is very toxic, as the Raindrop oils will begin the detox process immediately.

— *Doing Raindrop in Colorado*

## Lou Gehrig's Disease

I am sixty and have performed more than 120 Raindrop procedures and am a student working toward becoming a Naturopathic Doctor (ND). I have done a lot of facilitating the oils on family, saving a lot of doctor visits. We have seventeen grandchildren, and the children will always come to grandma for oils. I have lots of testimonies on our grandchildren, but there is one particular experience I want to share.

A lady came to me with Lou Gehrig's disease. She could hardly walk into the house. I had to help her get her jewelry and clothes off. She had a stomach tube and some paralysis of the throat. Her muscles twitched real bad in her back. I gave her a Raindrop.

The next time I saw her she told me that the next morning her voice was crystal clear. When I checked her back, her muscles were no longer twitching. I worked on her every other day for a month and then I advised her to go to the Young Living Clinic in Utah to finish the treatment. When she returned, she emailed me and said she was fine and that she loved going to the clinic.

My only disappointments were two ladies that really wanted help and were willing to accept Raindrop. But when they consulted with their doctors, they were advised against it and were told, "It would be the worst thing they could do for themselves."

— *Student Naturopath in Delaware*

## Raindrop on HIV Client

I have received Raindrop five times. it felt great but no perceivable improvement because I was already in great health. I just wanted to learn what it felt like so I could learn Raindrop Technique. I felt better afterwards, but was not ill beforehand. I have also done about 18 Raindrops, mostly on my kids and and friends, including one who regularly receives Raindrop because she was HIV positive. Very soothing to my children and loved ones.

— *Certified in Facial Rejuvenation from New York*

## Muscular Dystrophy

Used on myself, I felt a reduction of back pain and stress, and my energy level increased. It continued for about four days. Used on my thirteen-year-old son with muscular dystrophy, he felt comfortable and relaxed and was able to sleep through the night for the first time in months.

— *LSCC in New Jersey.*

## Raindrop on Horses

My clients, including horses, have all felt better after the technique was performed. Most people claim they feel like a weight has been lifted off of them, and they feel more clear and alert. Knowing the therapeutic grade oils have properties known to digest petrochemicals, this is my assumption, that they are feeling better due to the "cleaning" the oils do on a cellular level. Besides the after-effects, the animals and people feel very relaxed during the procedure, almost a meditative state. I plan to continue to perform this technique and teach others the benefit.

— *B.S. in Environmental Science from Illinois.*

## Thyroid Cancer

I had thyroid cancer, and in seven months, with colon cleansing, chinese wolfberry, and Raindrop Technique, the doctor couldn't find it any longer! I have since administered Raindrop Technique more than 200 times. I had two cases where the clients had loose stools the next day. One appreciated that fact since she had been constipated. The other was a vegetarian and surmised that the Raindrop was detoxifying her system. All others loved it, especially the hot towel at the end.

— *Licensed Massage Therapist and Esthetician, Florida*

## Relief with Scoliosis

I have exchanged RDTs with a friend approximately once a month over the past four years and have received it approximately 35 times. For my entire adult life I have had a pronounced amount of scoliosis. Additionally, the upper right quarter of my back has been very rounded with quite a lot of inflammation and stressed musculature due to thirty years of being a hairstylist. I have had regular chiropractic care and Rolfing treatments for a number of years, which have helped make these conditions less serious. However, within a few months of starting regular Raindrop treatments these chronic conditions began to improve well beyond the point I had been able to get to previously. Besides these very welcome benefits, I find RDT to be a deeply relaxing experience and have had no colds or flu in the last four years since starting Raindrop.

— *Hairstylist in Oregon*

## Shingles, Clogged Sinuses, and Fever

I have given about 47 Raindrops to various people and all of them benefited. A few were tired after the session and went home and slept for a few hours. In my opinion these individuals were detoxifying. During many sessions, my clients get so relaxed they fall asleep. Some specific example of my observations are as follows:

One client came in with shingles on lower lumbar area. After Raindrop a rash appeared in upper neck, right side of body (most likely virus leaving the spinal area). Used thyme and oregano on shingle area. Area heated up and was calmed down with mixing oil. After session client was very relaxed physically and mentally. She said she had come in irritated with her boyfriend, but after the session all irritation was gone.

A client came with her right sinus passage bothering her. After session her right sinus passage opened up. On another occasion the same client came in perspiring with a sinus infection and a fever of 99.5°F. After treatment her temperature went down to 98.7°F., her perspiring stopped, a lot of gas was relieved, and she stated she felt relaxed.

— *Certified Natural Health Practitioner and Colon Therapist, Maryland*

## Auto Accident

I was in pain from an auto accident. Stopped by to see a friend that was in town for a day or so. She had her oils with her. After listening to me about how bad my neck and head hurt she asked if she could rub her oils on my neck. She asked if I would mind the "smell" before she began. Needless to say I was in pain and willing to try anything. After the Raindrop treatment I was amazed at the relief I felt. I wanted some of these miracle oils. I am still using them and could not live without Valor™ and lavender. These I use every day. I also now do Raindrop Technique, myself.

Valor (one of the principal Raindrop oil blends) will get you through any situation. Before a speech I use a drop on the wrists and take a few deep breaths. Amazing difference. My friend lost her husband and I used it on her. It calmed her and helped her get through this sorrowful time. Another friend landed a job with a local radio station. He uses Valor to settle the nerves before going on the air. I could write a book on Valor. The Raindrop treatment is wonderful. Mine usually last up to three or more months. I use it on my husband also.

*— Loves Valor in North Carolina*

## Fighting Breast Cancer

As a recipient I have only just begun to experience Raindrop. (I have received it twice now.) I have been very pleased with the results so far. I am fighting a recurrence of breast cancer and feel that the oils have helped with the emotional upheaval I have felt. I intend to continue receiving the technique. I have had no skin reaction to any of the oils. And even the heat I was supposed to feel was not anywhere near as bad as the hot flashes I experience due to the medications I am taking. It was quite pleasant and very relaxing. I felt very good afterwards and for several hours even into the next day.

*— Hot Flashes from New Mexico*

## Rods in the Back

I have had four Raindrop sessions. I went to the grocery store right after the first session and was able to swing my hips side to side as never before. My back has two Herrington rods in with very little movement in frozen hips and shoulders previously.

*— Alberta, Canada*

## Daily Raindrop for MS

I have administered more than 50 Raindrop sessions. I personally felt very relaxed after the technique was applied to me. Most clients love the technique. It corrected scoliosis for one client. Another client has MS and the oils in RDT are being applied daily plus the other oils recommended for MS. This client has noticed an increase in strength and is sleeping much better.

— *Certified Massage Therapist, Indiana*

## Annual Raindrop for Scoliosis

I am a Licensed Massage Therapist and have a first degree scoliosis and often get chronic pain on the lengthened side near the vertebral border of my scapula. Immediately after my first Raindrop I no longer felt the discomfort that has been nagging me for years. The first treatment only left a "thumb print of discomfort," reminding me that something was there. This relief lasted nearly a year after just one Raindrop. Because of my occupation, the pain was beginning to resurface towards the end of the first year after I had received treatment. A year later (2000) I decided to get another Raindrop. Since the second treatment I no longer experience any aches or discomfort in that area. My back muscles and posture have improved and another Licensed Massage Therapist I know has mentioned that I have no signs of scoliosis any longer. I love the treatment because of its effectiveness. I plan to get another treatment this month (which will be my third annual Raindrop). Raindrop Technique has brought me positive results.

— *Licensed Massage Therapist in New York*

## Fewer Chiropractor Visits with Raindrop

I have received Raindrop about ten times now, and my scoliosis in the lumbar region of my back was greatly improved (straightened). My general health is improved when I have Raindrop Technique, as well as my state of mind. I have had some reddening of the skin during the procedure, but it goes away quickly and just tells me that it is working. My skin gets more red when I am not feeling well than when I am feeling well. My visits to the chiropractor are significantly reduced with Raindrop Technique.

— *Scoliosis in California*

## Spine Lengthens More than Two Inches

I have had scoliosis all of my adult life. I do not know about childhood as scoliosis screening was not available then. Along with the scoliosis came debilitating migraines. My first Raindrop came at a Level I class in Dallas with Dr. Gary Young. He had several doctors attending the class to take back measurements of those of us who had scoliosis and who were on the massage table getting ready to receive a Raindrop. The curvature of my spine at the top left measured out from the center one inch. After Raindrop, the doctors again took measurements. My spine had straightened and was no longer off by one inch. My spine had lengthened by 2.25 inches. I have since received forty Raindrops over a period of the last two-and-a-half years.

The headaches do not manifest as long as I use Raindrop on a regular basis. My whole body feels lighter after a Raindrop and no longer feels anxious and stressed mentally, emotionally, and physically. I carry a lot of stress at various points in my neck and shoulders. Using the oils releases the pain in these areas.

I have also found that by doing Raindrop on a regular basis, my immune system is much stronger. I have done more than 100 Raindrops at this time.

One Elder, on whom I performed Raindrop on a weekly basis, had severe pain from arthritis and spinal stenosis. He was in a wheelchair and could use a walker only with the greatest of assistance. I had his wife apply a blend of eucalyptus and melaleuca oils daily using the Raindrop Technique, which was in addition to his weekly Raindrop. Within a couple of weeks he was able to get himself out of his wheelchair, be pain free, and walk unassisted with his walker.

— *No Longer Anxious in New Jersey*

## Lymphoma

I had lymphoma and used RDT to help my immune system and general well-being while undergoing chemotherapy. When a painful bone marrow procedure was done in the spinal area, there were no after effects as compared to other patients in the same practice. The doctor was amazed at the lack of pain afterwards. I could walk, etc. I am now lymphoma free.

— *Naturopathic Doctor & Registered Massage Therapist, Texas*

## Benefited In Spite of Burn

I am a massage therapist and have received four Raindrops and administered three. My personal experiences were all positive and resulted in healing. I would definitely return for more. When I first started doing Raindrop I had no formal training, but learned it from a friend who had attended Young Living's Levels I and II. I had also read the *Essential Oils Desk Reference* and watched a video. The second time I used Raindrop on a friend the oils burned her neck area severely. Burn blisters developed. I had used too much oil. Because of that experience I did not use the therapy for a year or more until I received more indepth training. Even so, my friend felt that she had benefited from the technique and is willing to receive it again.
— *Certified, Licensed Massage Therapist from California*

## Why Did I Wait So Long?

I have done 20–30 Raindrops with a variety of responses, all good to one degree or another. One client reported her cold was gone in three days following a Raindrop. One got ill and vomited, possibly detoxing was my thinking. One developed a rash on her back and is a person that does NOT drink water and has poor dietary intake; my thought again is many toxins and not drinking enough water to flush them. I have seen feet become more in alignment following Raindrop and once watched a spine straighten up. I usually see some back redness from the oils—probably working on viruses. One client said, "Why did I wait so long to get one of these?"
— *Registered Nurse and Licensed Massage Therapist, Iowa*

## Low Back Pain and a Stiff Neck

I was having chronic lower back pain and a stiff neck. Massage gave some temporary relief, but it was never long lasting. After having one Raindrop application the stiffness in the neck was resolved. After having several Raindrops I found the lower back pain, which was always worse in the morning, was gone. I have had no unpleasant reactions from the oils except for a burning sensation on my neck, which was rapidly and completely relieved with the application of a massage oil to the area.
— *Back Pain Gone, Washington State*

## Severe Rash

I have experienced Raindrop Technique approximately 80 times. I would say that 70 of those experiences were pleasant, positive, and I felt better afterwards, both physically and emotionally. In ten of the experiences I detoxed severely, and my pain was worse. This lasted for 1-2 days each time, and then I was pain free. In these ten unpleasant experiences, I was also emotionally worse off, suffering from the temporary fear that RDT was not working.

I have now done about 20 Raindrops on others with 18 largely pleasant and positive experiences and two with only partially positive consequences. In general, with clients who had chronic pain, the RDT was very successful. However, in one case the client broke out in a severe rash the next day that covered her back, went under her arm pits, and stayed, weeping, draining, and itching, for two months. She stated that her chronic pain disappeared and stayed away, but the rash nearly drove her crazy.

Another client, heavily medicated for approximately seven years, showed immediate positive results but did not sleep that night and felt no better the next day. It is also noteworthy that her skin would not accept the oils. They merely sat on the skin with little or no absorption.

I would like to discuss my thoughts about the rash my client developed. I have seen what appears to be the same rash on patients in a hospital environment and, amazingly, recently, even myself. I treated it with hot water applications, drying with a blow dryer, and as much exposure to air as is possible. In addition, I applied an Aveeno Oatmeal Bath. I applied the oatmeal powder as a paste and also dry, as a powder. It stopped the rash from itching and prevented any further weeping. If I had known how well this works I could have had the client with the rash on her back soak in a hot oatmeal bath three times daily, use the hair dryer, and apply the dry powder in between. I do not suggest the topical application of any creams or ointments for such a rash. Experimenting on myself, I found these to make it worse.

— *An RN, RNP from Oregon*

## Concussion and Whiplash

I had both a head concussion and a whiplash injury within six months of each other. My first Raindrop re-aligned the spine and took pressure off the skull bones and the brain and removed the fear of injuring my head. At my second Raindrop my vertebrae sat one on top of the other in perfect alignment and there was no pressure anywhere in the bony structure of the body. It felt like a puppet on a string with the skull perfectly balanced. The energy flowed evenly and smoothly through the whole system. It was wonderful to experience. I have now had ten Raindrops and will continue to return for more.

— *Saskatchewan, Canada*

## Ankylosing Spondylitis

I was diagnosed with ankylosing spondylitis in 1990. ("Spondylitis" means inflammation of the spine while "ankylosing" means stiffness and inflexibility.) I researched and began to practice Raindrop in 2000. I found the treatment very soothing and comforting. Certainly the layering technique and the oils used result in a warm and penetrating sensation. Neither I nor my wife (on whom I performed the technique) ever had any negative indications from the technique.

After Raindrop, my back is much looser and more relaxed, and the pain level and stiffness have decreased measurably, as evidenced by my level of mobility. These are temporary benefits as far as I know, but the additional emotional relaxation and release are a welcome de-stressor as well.

— *Relaxed and Released in California*

## Asthma

I am actually filling this out for my now seven-year-old son who was in respiratory distress at the time of his first Raindrop treatment. He has a prior history of asthmatic episodes. The first time he had Raindrop done, he was on his second straight day of non-stop crouping during the course of a respiratory infection. He was to the point of exhaustion. The woman who did

Raindrop on him (on Christmas Eve of all times) really gave us a "Christmas Miracle." Following the Raindrop session, we brought our son home, put him in bed, and watched over him for the next four hours while he "slept it off." When he finally woke up, his croup was reduced to an occasional cough and he was coherent again. It was like the resurrection of Lazarus to us.

*— Lazarus in Michigan*

## Needed Emotionally Releasing Oils

I have had about 20 Raindrops since 1998. The first standard Raindrop I received I really didn't feel anything. I had no reactions on the skin or otherwise. It wasn't until my facilitator started using more of the emotional release oils did my body respond to the standard Raindrop oils. Since then I have received Raindrop treatments on a regular basis and consider it necessary for my physical and emotional maintenance and well-being. Since receiving some Raindrop training in 2000, I have done about 25 Raindrops on others. I have never had anyone say they felt worse or that they did not like it. Personally, I will never stop getting Raindrops. It has helped me and my loved ones to escape some pretty bad situations and conditions.

*— Excited About Raindrop in California*

## I Always Apply Them Neat

I am a Licensed Master Esthetician, an unlicensed Naturopath, and a Masseuse with twenty-five years experience. Since moving to Utah, I no longer practice naturopathy or massage as I used to do in Pennsylvania. My job now is as a wellness coordinator doing health screenings. A student introduced me to therapeutic-grade oils. I'd had worked with aromatherapy in private practice for about ten years at the time with minimal results. I was not enthusiastic when she first brought Young Living™ oils to my attention. Ten minutes after she applied Valor™ to my spine following a five-hour drive across the state, my attitude toward these oils changed, and I have used them ever since. I always apply them neat and have had no rash or injury. I have experienced an acute episode of diarrhea on a few occasions as the oils detoxify my system. I have Raindrop Technique done regularly by a local therapist and have received about 20 sessions so far.

*— Wellness Coordinator in Utah*

## Improved Eyesight

I have had Raindrop four times, and it improved my vision with the first session. I felt relaxed, with a feeling of peace and serenity. Other Raindrop sessions took pain away from my shoulder areas and assisted in the alignment of my spine. I have only had wonderful positive results from this technique.

— *Certified Reflexologist and Iridologist, Maryland*

## Help for Fibromyalgia

I had fibromyalgia and chronic fatigue and had been going downhill for seven years. Then I met someone who did Raindrop Technique. I was not healed, but I regained a considerable amount of my health that year. My Raindrops left me feeling like I was stronger and headed in the right direction. It relieved some of my pain. I would have had more therapies, but we moved and I was unable to find someone that knew the Raindrop Technique in my new city. The year that I received the treatments and used essential oils neat almost daily, my doctor told me that I had finally made great strides.

— *Looking for a Raindrop Facilitator in South Dakota*

## Chronic Skin Disorder Disappears

I have received about 20 RDTs myself and have done 40 or more on others. I have been involved with essential oils for some 20 years now and consider Raindrop to be a Godsend. I have fasted and used Raindrop with phenomenal benefits. My systems are operating at such a natural and authentic level with an energetic and wonderful sense of well being. I am 51. I used Raindrop on my son (24) who had some kind of lump about the size of a marble on his right forearm. I prayed as I applied each oil during the Raindrop. Afterwards, I was delighted to witness that there was no sign of any presence of the lump.

As a certified massage therapist, it is astounding to watch people get on the table with a dullness in their spirit and physical presence . . . then get up as a lit-up being. Not once has anyone complained of any problem with the Raindrop Technique. It is, as I have said before, a total Godsend and one of the only options available that can literally turn your health around.

I performed the Raindrop on a Malibu businessman who had been troubled with a skin disorder for some years. He had tried everything, even fasting, and could not get rid of it. He was self-conscious and did not like the response of women when they would look at his skin!

One Raindrop session with the man, and the skin condition was literally gone in less than a week. His twin reported to me that following the miracle, his brother's social life became much better and that his self-esteem also improved!

— *Massage Therapist in the Los Angeles Area.*

## Relief of Stress

I have received Raindrop Technique once. What I experienced was a most incredible experience. I had an awful lot of stress in my life at the time and the technique relaxed me physically and emotionally. It gave me such a sense of peacefulness and relaxation. I would love to do it again and would definitely recommend it to anyone.

— *Peace and Relaxation from Washington State*

## The Common Cold

I had a bad cold, and a friend offered to do the Raindrop Technique. My cold was gone in two days, which is a lot shorter time than most of the colds I have ever had.

— *Cured of Cold in California*

## Chronic Pain from Accidents and Sports Injuries

I have received Raindrop eight times and have given it to clients about 20 times. I have had many clients who have felt very energized after a Raindrop. One client in particular has suffered from a lot of chronic pain on a daily basis due to car accidents and sports injuries. He has headaches almost daily. After his first Raindrop he was pain-free for a whole day. Two weeks later he received another Raindrop and was pain-free for several days.

Personally I have had good, pleasant Raindrops, as well as Raindrops that resulted in nausea and vomiting of mucous. Regardless, I always feel that I have benefited from them.

— *Raindrop Practitioner from Iowa*

## Fractured Neck Vertebrae

I have performed RDT about ten times. One person who had had fractured vertebrae in her neck due to a car accident in 1996 was given a Raindrop recently. She had not had any treatments for the last two years and had just begun to return to treatment. She was seen one time by a chiropractor just prior to the Raindrop who found her legs out of balance, one being two inches longer than the other. On her next visit to the chiropractor after receiving the Raindrop, the doctor found a significant improvement in the balance of her legs. There was over an inch of improvement. One leg is now less than one inch longer than the other.
— *Licensed Clinical Sound Worker from Colorado*

## Pain of Fibromyalgia Subsides

I have been in pain from fibromyalgia for fifteen plus years taking drugs every few hours. Five years ago I finally found a doctor who would take me off the drugs and prescribe acupuncture. At one point I was also going to a chiropractor four times a week. I felt like the rest of my life was going to be lived on the couch. About nine months ago I discovered Raindrop and essential oils. When I get the Raindrop I feel so relaxed and calm. The pain in my neck and shoulders and joints has subsided greatly. When I overdo it, I can't wait to get the next Raindrop because I know how good it makes me feel, and without taking drugs!
— *No Longer Living on the Couch in Texas*

## Neuropathy in the Feet and Toes

I am not a licensed practitioner and only teach people to do RDT with a partner or trade with friends. The most noticeable change I have witnessed after giving a Raindrop session was from a woman who mentioned she had a rather severe amount of neuropathy (lack of feeling in her limbs and feet) which she had had for a few years. As she got off the table and started to put on her shoes she stopped and, in a rather amazed voice, said she could feel the carpet under her toes. She said she couldn't remember the last time she felt that sensation.

I have performed the technique approximately 70 times, all of which were reported as pleasant by the receiver. I have had no reports of any kind of negative impact except for the six or seven people who had headaches afterwards and who had not drunk sufficient water following the procedure.

— *Trading for Raindrops in Oregon*

## Lyme Disease

I have always used oils neat on myself since I found them. After years of upper body pain and difficulty breathing I was diagnosed with fibromyalgia, Lyme disease and stress. Since using the oils I rarely have had pain or a hard time getting a full breath. I have received two Raindrops, and both times it was by someone who was brand new at doing it. I still had positive results. I am hoping others in my area will desire to practice this so I can receive more treatments. It's terrific.

— *Relieved in Michigan*

## Scoliosis as an Emotional Issue

I have congenital scoliosis with a large curve below the waistline and a compensating curve at the top. I was given Raindrop approximately once a month for well over a year and less frequently after that. Only once during the monthly sessions did my back straighten out almost perfectly, but it slowly curved again. The problem was that I was not receiving them frequently enough, or so I thought.

About a year ago, during a YLEO Level II training in Idaho, I had a profound emotional healing which has changed my attitude to myself, my self-esteem, and my ability to support myself both emotionally and financially. During the year that followed I received two Raindrops, one in January and one in October. These Raindrops were done by the same person as when I was having them once a month. Nothing she did changed, but I had changed. My back, before she started, was already so straight she was in awe. Of course I cannot see it, but she says the almost two-inch curve at the bottom is now less than 3/4 inch. I believe her because I can stand at work all day without pain now and if I run my fingers down my back, they do not swerve enough for me to notice a swerve anymore. I have "before" x-rays but not any "after" x-rays yet. I am not in a hurry for an x-ray so I will wait until I am even straighter or need one.

— *British Columbia, Canada*

## Avoided Surgery with Scoliosis

I have been doing Raindrop since 1997 and have performed it more than 60 times. I have seen dramatic results with some of my clients.

I have had six clients that had scoliosis so bad they were facing surgery. One client, after the first session, could straighten up. Within a week she found she could be in certain positions without discomfort for the first time. Another client, after three sessions, went back to her doctor and she didn't need surgery.

The net result was out of six cases that were scheduled for surgery to correct their posture, not one needed the surgery after Raindrop. I have found in most cases of scoliosis (about 70%) that there is some relief from Raindrop for the recipient, either very subtle or a dramatic experience.
— *Raindrop Practitioner in New York*

## Received Raindrop While Pregnant

I have had many viruses in my life, in my eyes, Bell's palsy, and a few that even the doctors couldn't peg. So when I received my first Raindrop at a convention I knew that my spine would probably heat up when the oregano was applied as I know that I do have viruses and fungus along my spine. However, I did not need any mixing oil to be applied as the burn was not unpleasant. The rest of my first Raindrop was very pleasant. Afterwards I had a headache and didn't feel spectacular so I went to bed quite early. The following morning I felt fine and enjoyed the rest of the convention.

Two months later I was at a Raindrop training in Phoenix and was again receiving another treatment (my second). This time my back did not heat up at all with any of the oils, including oregano, and I had no headache afterwards. I felt that I benefited greatly from just even one treatment!

I would like to point out that for both of these Raindrops I was pregnant. I was only willing to receive these Raindrops using the high quality, therapeutic grade oils of Young Living and not any other ones. Shortly after this meeting we saw the baby via ultrasound and he appeared very healthy.

Our baby boy was born March 7, 2002. The labor was easy and my son is super healthy, no problems. We use oils on him and his three-year-old brother all the time applied neat (i.e. without dilution). I cannot remember the last time that I have been sick (seriously) since using the oils

during the last three years, and my two boys are the picture of health. My husband is a welder and his back gets really tight. After Raindrop he feels great and his back knots go away. He is always asking me to do another one. My experiences doing Raindrop on others have been 100% positive.
— *A Mother and Wife from Alberta, Canada*

## Relief for Fibromyalgia Pain

I had my first two Raindrops in May and June, and it helped reduce, almost completely, the pain I had from fibromyalgia. I have not had the fibromyalgia pain since. I have also stopped drinking sodas and have greatly limited my coffee intake, too. I had my next treatments in November, and they were absolutely wonderful, helping to really relax my muscles, which tend to be very tight.
— *Registered Nurse in Arizona*

## High Fever

Raindrop is one of the most profound therapies I have ever experienced. It makes you feel so good and puts you into a state of relaxation. In January 2000 I had just come home from a Raindrop training workshop and my six-year-old daughter had a fever. I gave her a Raindrop that day. Her fever was 102° before. After I finished she had a completely normal body temperature, which stayed that way. During the Raindrop on my daughter I used oregano and thyme neat and then put mixing oil on to stop any itching she was experiencing. I feel the Raindrop saved her from the virus she had in her body that day.
— *A Mother from Kentucky*

## Has Received Raindrop More than Eighty Times

I cannot speak highly enough for Raindrop treatment. I have received it more than 80 times since 1998. I had a number of diseases that caused toxins to stay in my system, in my spine and neck. The treatment each time caused the toxins to be moved out of the tissues and spinal column, which were then eliminated out of my system in the following days. In the early stages it was necessary for me to rest the next day after the Raindrop and drink lots of water, but this was only because of the toxins moving to be eliminated out of my body.

I am 100% healed and consider the Raindrop treatment one of the main contributions to this success along with the use of supplements and change of diet. The treatments have always left me feeling a major positive shift in my body. There is no way I would have the good heath I have today without receiving this technique on a continual basis.

— *100% Healed in California*

### Scoliosis in Child

I am not a licensed health care professional, but have been doing Raindrop Technique since 1999. One client, a child (age 13), had an almost complete reversal of scoliosis after receiving RDT for a period of six months. I trained her mom and assisted her with the first two sessions. As for me personally, I am in good health in general, and, although I always felt better after a Raindrop, I saw no other change except that one of the sessions relieved the pain of an old neck injury.

— *Raindrop Practitioner in North Carolina*

### Would Have Raindrop Every Day If I Could

Physically I feel much better and healthier after each Raindrop. As a result, I am definitely more grounded, clear, and calm. I had a potentially very emotionally-charged interaction after one of the Raindrops and was in a remarkable state of calm, patience, and receptivity, unlike at any other time under the same emotional-relational circumstances.

I would have a RDT every day of the week if I could. I have had absolutely no, none, nil, zilch negative reactions; nil skin reactions. And I have been applying therapeutic grade essential oils neat (undiluted) on and in myself and my children and my husband for 3.5 years with no, none, nil, zilch negative reactions. We are all in greater physical and emotional states.

— *None, Nil and Zilch from California*

### Various Infections Cleared Up

I had a viral infection when receiving my first Raindrop. The fever, headache, and earache were all gone in one day and the infection completely disappeared in two days.

Some time later, when I received my second Raindrop, I had another infection. Following the Raindrop my sore throat disappeared overnight, an ear infection disappeared the next day, and the fever, headache, and pains disappeared in one-and-a-half days.

I did a Raindrop on a client with a yeast infection, and it cleared up in two days. I did a Raindrop on a leukemia patient with a urinary tract infection, and the UTI cleared up in about a week after the Raindrop.

— *Raindrop Practitioner in Missouri*

## Back Strain and Sciatica

My sister strained her back and was in a lot of pain. She was afraid she would be laid up for weeks. After one Raindrop treatment from me she felt a lot better. After only a couple of days her back was free of pain.

My neighbor has a herniated disk, and the sciatic nerve gives him a lot of pain down his leg. After his first Raindrop treatment, he reported that he was able to sleep better that night than he had in weeks.

— *Sister and Neighbor in California*

## Brain Injury

I have a son (18 yrs) who became extremely ill two years ago. The medical community didn't have any answers or solutions as to why the myelin sheath was destroyed in large areas of his brain. He suffered brain injury and loss of the use of his entire right side. He also lost memory, has double vision, and some hearing loss. I have been using the oils on him without diluting them (neat) every day on his feet and have done the Raindrop six times on him. I've never seen a bad reaction, but I have seen some wonderful improvements. He loves it. I have had several others tell me they notice an improvement in him.

— *Mother in Michigan*

## Flu Symptoms

I have had two Raindrops. In both instances I felt I was beginning to get flu symptoms. After Raindrop there were no more symptoms. So I was able to continue to go to work and lead a healthy life, relieved that I was not ill.

— *Healthy Life in California*

# Discussion & Conclusion

As stated in the questionnaire that forms the basis for this study, "this is not a precision survey, but a general determination survey." The intent was to compile a sample of experiences from doing and receiving Raindrop Technique that would lend itself to a certain amount of statistical summarizing while soliciting verbal commentaries that would provide insight into the practice and outcomes of Raindrop that cannot be conveyed by mere figures. I believe these objectives were accomplished. I believe that if anyone were to conduct a similar survey from a similar population, they would obtain similar, if not essentially the same, results.

As for the 74 commentaries listed on pages 21–49, they are anecdotal only. To have any medical validity they would all have to have been under some form of medical control and verification. This would have been a prohibitive expense in compiling such a variety of information. Even so, just because they are unverified, subjective, and anecdotal does not mean they have no research value.

All information is valuable if not interpreted beyond its foundation. In this instance, these stories and anecdotes represent a true sample of what receivers and facilitators think and believe about Raindrop. In that context, this is valid science the same as any opinion poll is a valid form of gathering data of a subjective nature.

The data and experiences compiled in this study do not provide scientific proof that Raindrop has any specific benefits or risks. However, this study does provide a strong body of evidence that Raindrop is thought by the vast majority of its participants to benefit people in ways both objective and subjective, physical and emotional, social and spiritual.

The beginning of science in any new field starts with collections of anecdotes. From such collections, hypotheses are conceived. From such hypotheses, experiments are designed and carried out. From the results of such experiments, theories are developed and put to the scientific test again and again until they are refined and expressed as laws of nature.

This is the first study ever to be published on Raindrop Technique. The content of this publication is fertile with many ideas for additional research and can serve as a starting point for future studies of a more rigorous nature.

This research serves many purposes. For those who wish to consider whether to receive and/or to practice Raindrop, this work enables a more informed choice than was heretofore possible. It also provides a basis for hospital administrators, health care professionals, aromatherapists, legislators, regulatory boards, and others to consider whether they should seriously explore the utility of this technique or not. It also provides a basis for the health care insurance industry to consider reimbursement for Raindrop services as a valid modality for health and wellness.

The anecdotes reported here are based on more than 14,000 experiences in Raindrop from the perspectives of both receivers and facilitaters. As such, these accounts offer a great deal of insight and wisdom into the actual daily practice of Raindrop that should be a valuable education for all who practice or aspire to practice Raindrop Technique.

And if the safety and/or the efficacy of Raindrop is a question, these data clearly outline the boundaries of these issues. To those who engage in it, Raindrop Technique is safe. Raindrop Technique is effective.

# Bibliography

1. Higley, Connie, and Higley, Alan. (2001) *Reference Guide for Essential Oils*, revised edition, Abundant Health, Olathe, Kansas. 497 pp.
2. Manwaring, Brian, editor. (2001) *Essential Oils Desk Reference*, second edition, Essential Science Publishing Company, Orem, Utah. 461 pp.
3. Burroughs, Stanley, (1993) *Healing for the Age of Enlightenment*, sixth edition, Burroughs Books, Reno, Nevada. 149 pp.
4. Decker, Robert, & Sheldon, Gary, (1985) *The Body Electric*. William Morrow Publishers, New York, NY. 324 pp.
5. Cary, Francis A., (2000) *Organic Chemistry*, fourth edition, McGraw-Hill, Boston, Mass. 1108 pp.
6. Pénoël, Daniel, and Pénoël, Rose-Marie, (1998) *Natural Home Health Care Using Essential Oils, Introduction of the Theory, Practice, and Technique of Integral Aromatherapy (Osmobiosis)*, Osmobiose Publishing, La Drome, France. 236 pp.
7. Pert, Candace, (1999) *Molecules of Emotion*, Touchstone edition, Simon & Schuster, New York, NY. 368 pp.
8. Price, Shirley, and Price, Len, (1999) *Aromatherapy for Health Professionals*, second edition. Foreword by Daniel Pénoël, MD, Churchill-Livingston, London, England. 391 pp.
9. Schnaubelt, Kurt, (1995) *Advanced Aromatherapy: The Science of Essential Oil Therapy*, translated by J. Michael Beasley, Healing Arts Press, Rochester, Vermont. 138 pp.
10. Schnaubelt, Kurt, (1999) *Medical Aromatherapy: Healing with Essential Oils*, Frog Ltd., Berkeley, California. 296 pp.
11. Valnet, Jean, (1990) *The Practice of Aromatherapy*, edited by Robert Tisserand, Healing Arts Press, Rochester, Vermont. 279 pp.
11. Williams, David G. (1997) *Essential Oil Chemistry: An Introduction for Aromatherapists, Beauticians, Retails, and Students*, Michelle Press, Dorset, England. 334 pp.
12. Young, D. Gary. (1996) *Aromatherapy: The Essential Beginning*. second edition. Essential Press Publishing, Salt Lake City, UT. 174 pp.

# Appendix A:
# Raindrop Survey Questionnaire

The following questionnaire was sent out on eight email chat lines in October, November, and December, 2001. It was also copied and sent by ordinary postal service to many others not on the chat lines.

In order to encourage free and candid responses, the confidentiality of the respondents was assured to those submitting completed questionnaires. In the questionnaire, itself, only the country, state or province, and gender were requested as identifying demographics. However, that does not mean the respondents are unknown or untraceable. In all but a few (less than 0.5%) an email or postal address is known. In most cases the name of the respondent is also known. These confidential data are part of the permanent file of original data collected for this project by the Center for Aromatherapy Research and Education. Hence, any specific respondent could be contacted if there was a good reason for doing so.

The original survey fit on two 8.5" x 11" pages with space allowed for answers. In this appendix the content of the questionnaire is presented in a reconfigured format to fit the page size of this publication but is otherwise a verbatim account. The cover letter that accompanied the survey is also reproduced here:

## Raindrop Survey Cover Letter

Dear Friends:

The Center for Aromatherapy Research and Education (CARE) is compiling data on Raindrop Technique outcomes to provide a research basis for its application. We need lots of respondents to gain the statistical numbers needed to make a valid study.

We will publish the results of this effort on this chat line, as well as elsewhere. While the tone of this first effort is general and would be considered as "soft science," it is nevertheless an effort to compile something of a statistical and objective nature about Raindrop. Between all of us, there must be thousands of experiences with Raindrop.

Everything will be private and confidential. I am not even asking for your names unless you want to volunteer them. If you mail, email, or fax your information, your return mail or call information will be there for me if I need to contact you for any clarifications or questions.

The results will be useful to all of us who, from time to time, are asked for data or scientific studies to support the claims made for Raindrop, as well as information on any untoward effects experienced by some. The more data I receive, the greater will be the validity of the study.

Thanks so much
David Stewart, Ph.D.
Executive Director, CARE, Inc.

## Raindrop Technique Outcome Research Questionnaire
Center for Aromatherapy Research and Education (CARE)
Rt. 4, Box 646, Marble Hill, MO 63764
• (573) 238-4846• <careclasses@raindroptraining.com> •

BEFORE YOU BEGIN, PLEASE READ INSTRUCTIONS AT THE END OF THIS QUESTIONNAIRE

1. Country _____
   State or Province_____
   Gender_____

### FOR RAINDROP RECEIVERS

2. In what year did you first receive a Raindrop?_____
3. Estimate how many times you have received Raindrop since (and including) your first_____

4. Evaluate your experience(s) following receipt of a Raindrop by estimating  the number of experiences for the following categories. Do the best you can in recalling. This is not a precision survey, but a general determination survey. Check as many as appropriate.

   Positive_____        Neutral_____        Negative_____

   Pleasant_____        Neutral_____        Unpleasant_____

   Resulted in a healing_____
           No perceptible results_____
                   Caused harm or injury_____
   Felt better afterwards_____
           No change in feeling_____
                   Felt worse afterwards_____
   State of health improved_____
           No change in health_____
                   General health got worse_____

Emotional state improved_____
        No change in emotions_____
                Emotional state worsened_____
Would receive it again_____
        Maybe so, maybe not_____
                Would never receive it again_____

5.  Please explain your answers or give a testimonial of what Raindrop did for you, positive or negative. Write on the back of this sheet or use additional sheets as needed. Your full and candid answers will be greatly appreciated. Remember everything is confidential. Your identity will never be revealed.

## For Raindrop Facilitators

6.  In what year did you first perform a Raindrop on someone?

        _____

7.  Estimate how many times have you performed Raindrop since (and including) your first? _____

8.  Evaluate your experiences with clients receiving Raindrop by estimating numbers of cases (or percents of your total) for the following categories. Do the best you can in recalling. This is not a precision survey, but a general determination survey.

    Positive_____         Neutral_____         Negative_____

    Pleasant_____         Neutral_____         Unpleasant_____

    Resulted in a healing_____
            No perceptible results_____
                    Caused harm or injury_____
    Felt better afterwards_____
            No change in feeling_____
                    Felt worse afterwards_____

State of health improved_____
    No change in health_____
        General health got worse_____
Emotional state improved_____
    No change in emotions_____
        Emotional state worsened_____
Would receive it again_____
    Maybe so, maybe not_____
        Would never receive it again_____

9.  Please elaborate on your answers or give selected accounts of what Raindrop has done for your clients, in general, either positive or negative. Write on the back of this sheet or use additional sheets as needed. Your full and candid answers will be greatly appreciated. Remember everything is confidential. Your identity will never be revealed.

10. How were you trained to do Raindrop Technique? (choose one or more)
    * Personally Trained one-on-one or in a small group by Dr. Gary Young_____
    * Trained at a Young Living Level I Program_____
    * Trained by someone who took the YL Level I Program_____
    * Educational Institution other than YL_____
      Name of Institution_____
    * Learned from a book_____
      Title of Book_____
    * Learned from a video_____
      Title of Video_____
    * Other_____

11. What Brand of Oils did you use in doing Raindrop?
    * Exclusively Young Living Oils_____
    * Occasionally use other brands, but mostly use Young Living_____
    * Occasionally use Young Living, but mostly use other brands_____
    * Usually use brands other than Young Living_____
      Other brands I use_____

12. Are you a licensed professional? (yes or no)_____
    If yes, specify what type or types such as DC, ND, OD, RN, OMD,
    MD, LMT, CMT, PT, etc. _____

    • Feel free to add any comments you would like to include as
      additional information.

END OF QUESTIONNAIRE

THANK YOU FOR YOUR PARTICIPATION

INSTRUCTIONS:  The information to be compiled from these
questionnaires is for statistical research purposes only. No names or
addresses, whether US postal or email, will not be given out to anyone.
The results of the survey will be published on the chat line from which
you receive this questionnaire.

Your cooperation and assistance in this project is greatly appreciated.
A prompt response is necessary inasmuch as we want to complete this
tabulation by December 15th Questionnaires received after that date
may not be included in the tally.

YOU MAY BE BOTH A RAINDROP RECEIVER AND
FACILITATOR. COMPLETE ALL QUESTIONS
THAT PERTAIN TO YOU.

Please mail to Care at the address on p. 1, or fax to CARE at
(573) 238-2010, or email it to CARE at careclasses@raindroptraining.com.
To respond via email we don't need the form with the questions; just write
numbers 1 thru 12 and your answers corresponding to the questions.

# Index of Conditions Reported by Respondents
## Compiled by Judy Addington, LMT, CR, SCCI

Ancylosing spondulitis 40
Antibiotics 31
Arthritis 37
Asthma 40
Auto accident pain (neck, head) 35

Back pain 24, 25, 27, 29, 31, 32, 33, 38, 41, 49
Bell's Palsy 28, 46
Brain injury 49
Bronchitis 32

Chronic fatigue 42
Chronic pain 39, 43
Chronic skin disorder 42
Circulation 22
Cold feet 22
Colds 29, 31, 34, 38, 43
Concussion 40

Detox 26, 31, 32, 33, 38, 39, 41, 45, 46, 48
Dowager's Hump 31

Ear infection 49
Emotionally uplifting 23, 24, 26, 30, 32, 41, 45, 46, 48
Epstein-Barr 27

Fever 34, 47
Fibromyalgia 42, 44, 45, 47
Flu 29, 34, 49

Headache 27, 37, 43
Herniated disc 30, 49
Horses 33

Leg length 44
Lou Gehrig's disease 32

Lump on arm 42
Lyme disease 45
Lymphoma 37

Multiple Sclerosis (MS) 36
Muscle pain 29, 34
Muscular dystrophy 33

Neck pain 48
Negative reactions 23, 30, 31, 39
Nerves 35
Neuropathy 44
Night sweats 22

Plantar fascitis 23
Pregnant 46

Quadriplegic 22

Rash 23, 39

Sciatic pain 28, 29, 49
Scoliosis 22, 25, 27, 28, 29, 30, 34, 36, 37, 45
Shingles 34
Sinun infection 31, 34
Sleep 23, 25, 27, 33, 36
Sore throat 49
Spinal meningitis 27
Stiff hips/shoulders 35, 42

Thyroid cancer 33

Viral infection 48
Vision 42

Whiplash 27, 40
Wrist pain 31

Yeast infection 49